Save Your Life
With
Basic Baking Soda

*Becoming pH Balanced
In an Unbalanced World*

Blythe Ayne, PhD

Save Your Life
With
Basic Baking Soda

Becoming pH Balanced
In an Unbalanced World

Blythe Ayne, PhD

Save Your Life With
Basic Baking Soda

Becoming pH Balanced in an Unbalanced World
Blythe Ayne, Ph.D.

Emerson & Tilman, Publishers
129 Pendleton Way #55
Washougal, WA 98671

The ***How to Save Your Life*** series:
Save Your Life with the Dynamic Duo: Vitamins D3 & K2
Save Your Life with the Phenomenal Lemon & Lime
Save Your Life with Awesome Apple Cider Vinegar
Save Your Life with the Power of pH Balance
Save Your Life with the Elixir of Water
Save Your Life with Stupendous Spices

www.BlytheAyne.com

ebook ISBN: 978-1-957272-47-4
Paperback ISBN: 978-1-957272-48-1
Hardbound ISBN: 978-1-957272-49-8
Large Print ISBN: 978-1-957272-50-4
Audiobook ISBN: 978-1-957272-51-1

[1. HEALTH & FITNESS/Diet & Nutrition/Nutrition
2. HEALTH & FITNESS/Healing
3. HEALTH & FITNESS/Diseases/General]
BIC: FM
First Edition

Table of Contents:

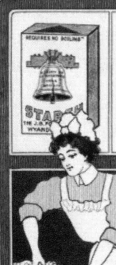
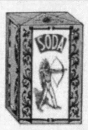
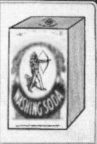

Baking Soda

means delicious soda biscuits, and other things which can be made only at their best with Wyandotte Baking Soda.

Starch

will make all starched things, such as shirts, shirt-waists and aprons, easier to iron, and look better when they are ironed.

Washing Soda

will make your clothes and table linen whiter and daintier with less work than any other washing compound.

Chapter 1
What is Sodium Bicarbonate aka, Baking Soda?

*I*t *Has a Few Aliases!*

Baking soda also goes by:

Sodium bicarbonate

Bicarbonate of soda

Sodium hydrogen carbonate

Sodium acid carbonateSodium hydrogen carbonate
Vichy salt

It's found in nahcolite deposits

Which are also called thermokalite

There will *not* be a test. But isn't it interesting all the names this simple household product has accrued?

Found in Evaporated Lake Basins

Sodium bicarbonate, more commonly called baking soda, is a white crystalline solid with a slightly salty taste due to its low alkaline pH of between 8-9.5. Its chemical formula is $NaHCO_3$, noting its composition of sodium ions and bicarbonate ions.

The most natural form of sodium bicarbonate is nahcolite, a mineral found all around the world, but primarily mined in California, Colorado, Wyoming, Utah, Botswana, and Kenya, with significant deposits in Uganda, Turkey, and Mexico.

Nahcolite, also called thermokalite, forms in the reaction of carbon dioxide with the mineral trona in evaporated lake basins.

But sodium bicarbonate is also manufactured in the human body! Among its many duties, it helps maintain the pH balance of the blood, it contributes to carrying carbon dioxide from the body's tissues to the lungs to be expelled, it helps neutralize stomach acids, and also helps neutralize arterial plaque acids.

Basic Baking Soda

The title, **Save Your Life with Basic Baking Soda**, is a play on the word, "basic." Baking soda is a base/basic, alkaline substance, and it's also basic in our daily lives.

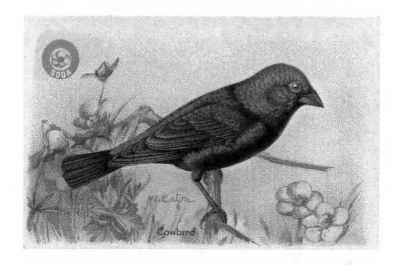

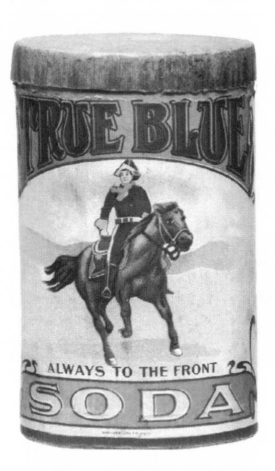

Chapter 2
Baking Soda – A Brief History

The "Rise" of Baking Soda

Sodium bicarbonate has been used by humans for over 5,000 years.

Ancient Egyptians used natron, a natural mixture of sodium carbonate decahydrate and sodium carbonate, to make soap, to brush their teeth, apply to wounds, to make glass ornaments and vessels, as a component in the paint they made for their hieroglyphics, and in mummification. The natron was recovered from dry lake-bed deposits or extracted from the ashes of plants by burning seaweed and other marine plants.

The Romans used soda ash for making glass, baking bread, and medicinal purposes.

Since the Middle Ages, bakers used carbonates as leaveners to lighten and raise batter due to the release of carbon dioxide, which bubbles up when dissolved in water or an acidic product, such as sour milk, is added.

Historically, Arabs cooked with wood ash or potash, also known as potassium carbonate, to produce leavening. This process was unknown to Europeans until the eighteenth century. Water-rinsed wood ashes, known as pearlash, were used to make cakes if the recipe included an acidic ingredient, but it left an unpleasant aftertaste.

Meanwhile, wood sources were diminishing. So in 1775, the French Academy of Sciences ran a contest with the goal of discovering a tastier alternative.

Nicolas LeBlanc, a French chemist, finally won the contest in 1791, by producing sodium carbonate, also known as soda ash. But his method of producing soda ash from salt and sulfuric acid still contained potash, which continued to have a bitter flavor.

The method of producing baking soda from the union of the metal, sodium, and carbonic acid, white in color with a brackish flavor, was discovered in 1801 by Professor Sigismund Friedrcih Hermbstaedt (1760-1833) and Valentin Rose, the Younger (1762-1807), a German chemist and apothecary, at the *Collegium Medico-chirurgicum* in Berlin.

Sodium Bicarbonate as a Leavening Agent

Although baking soda was imported from England to America during colonial times, it wasn't until 1839 that it was produced in the United States.

Then, in 1846, Austin Church, a Connecticut physician, and John Dwight, a farmer from Massachusetts, established a factory in New York to manufacture baking soda.

Dr. Church's son, John, owned *Vulcan Spice Mills,* with an an arm and hammer logo representing Vulcan, the Roman god of fire and forge. The new baking soda company adopted the still universally recognized *Arm & Hammer* logo.

But, it wasn't until 1861when Belgian industrial chemist, Ernest Solvay, developed the Solvay process, that industrial-scale production of baking soda became possible. The Solvay process plants were producing most of the world's soda ash by the 1890s.

In 1938 the entire picture was changed. Large deposits of the mineral, trona, were discovered near the Green River in Wyoming, also reaching to Utah and Colorado, from which sodium carbonate could be extracted more cheaply than produced by the Solvay process.

Saleratus

The word "saleratus," from Latin meaning, "aerated salt," was first used in the nineteenth century, referring to both potassium bicarbonate and sodium bicarbonate.

Saleratus appears in Rudyard Kipling's novel, *Captains Courageous,* in reference to the product being used extensively in commercial fishing to prevent freshly-caught fish from spoiling.

And from the notes for **Little House on the Prairie,** here is a list of the amounts of some of the food products pioneers were recommended to carry for each person traveling west in a covered wagon:

200 pounds of flour

30 pounds of pilot bread (hardtack)

10 pounds of rice

5 pounds of coffee

2 pounds of tea

25 pounds of sugar

1/2 bushel of dried beans

1 bushel of dried fruit

2 pounds of saleratus (baking soda)

10 pounds of salt

1/2 bushel of cornmeal

1/2 bushel of corn, parched and ground

1 small keg of vinegar

"Saleratus was made by pouring water through wood ashes, producing lye. The lye was then evaporated by boiling, leaving a residue called black salt. The salt was purified by fire, resulting in potash. Further baking in a kiln caused all the carbon impurities to be burned off, changing the potash into pearlash, which was fermented, producing carbonic acid that was then absorbed by the pearlash. The rendered solid was heavier, whiter, and drier than the pearlash, and had finally become saleratus."

http://www.pioneergirl.com/blog/archives/4146

(Now, doesn't that make one wonder who imagined that pouring water through the fireplace ashes would result in something to put into the ingredients for making bread?)

In 1927, the *Journal of Chemical Education* observed that baking soda could be used to prevent the common cold by keeping an alkaline balance in the body, with doses of sodium bicarbonate, along with small quantities of calcidine and iodine.

Now we know that not only does baking soda have antibacterial properties, but that it can alter bacterial susceptibility to antibiotics by targeting the *proton motive force* (the force created by the transfer of protons or electrons across a membrane, which can then be used for chemical, mechanical, or osmotic processes)—making it a potential new weapon in the race against antibiotic resistance.

Baking soda is on the World Health Organization's list of essential medicines.

A 2002 United Nations Environment Programme (UNEP) publication reported that the majority of sodium bicarbonate global applications were in human and animal food, with only about five percent of its use in cosmetics.

Today, "natural soda ash" refined from the mineral trona, a non-marine evaporite mineral, is the standard regarding quality and purity, processed from sodium-carbonate-bearing brines.

The Green River Basin of Wyoming, Utah, and Colorado, is the world's largest naturally-occurring trona area, mined as the primary source of sodium carbonate in the United States. It has replaced the Solvay process used in most of the rest of the world to produce sodium carbonate.

Today, this chemical powerhouse is produced globally, with an estimated volume of two million tons per year.

Chapter High Points:

1. Ancient Egyptians used the base of baking soda, na-tron, for everything from soap, to toothpaste, to paints used in their hieroglyphics, to mummifica-tion.

2. Different forms of carbonates were used in baking throughout history, each with its own flavor draw-back.

3. In 1846, Austin Church and John Dwight estab-lished a baking soda factory in New York. Its logo employed Church's son's mill logo, the readily rec-ognizable arm and hammer, representing the god Vulcan.

4. In 1861, Ernest Solvay develop the Solvay System for producing baking soda.

5. In 1938, large deposits of trona were discovered near the Green River in Wyoming and crossing sev-eral states. Sodium carbonate, from which soda bi-carbonate is produced, is readily extracted from these deposits.

6. Saleratus is a nineteenth-century word for sodium bicarbonate.

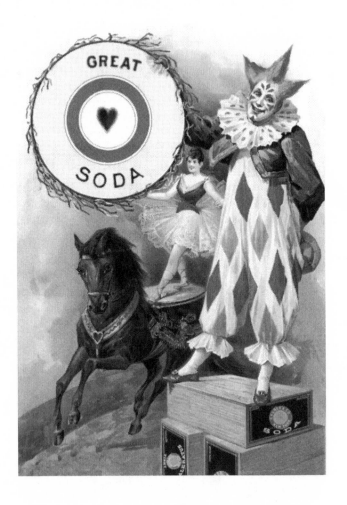

Chapter 3
Baking and Cooking with Baking Soda

A mong its many talents, baking soda is a leavening agent to make baked goodies such as bread, croissants, cakes, muffins, cupcakes, pancakes, and so forth. Whatever needs to rise!

When baking soda is combined with an acidic ingredient such as sour milk, molasses, lemon juice, etc., the resulting raising action is a process of carbon dioxide gas (CO_2) being released, expanding in the heat of the oven, and absorbed by the combined ingredients' cells, thus causing the protein in the batter to become fluffy and yet firm, and creating the delicious raised, leavened, product.

A Few Tips

In the realm of cooking, baking soda is used primarily for leavening baked goods. But it can also be used when baking vegetables to give them a heightened, attractive color.

Beans

Add a sprinkle of baking soda to the water of soaking dried beans. Beans contain a type of sugar called oligosaccharides, which can produce gas and a bloated feeling. Oligosaccharides make it all the way to the large intestine before being fully digested, and this can cause the production of gas. Adding a teaspoon of baking soda per cup of dried beans to the soaking beans reduces the oligosaccharides.

Secondly, the alkaline component of baking soda causes the pectin to break down into smaller molecules. The beans will cook faster, and have improved texture.

Starchy Veggies

Like beans, starchy vegetables such as potatoes and cassava also benefit from boiling in baking soda. When the baking soda softens the pectin, it loosens starch granules in the vegetables, and this makes for a softer texture.

Caramel and Baking Soda

When making caramel from sugar or caramelizing milk, add an eighth of a teaspoon of baking soda to the caramel. The sugars will rapidly turn brown and develop a nutty caramel aroma.

Coffee and Tea and Baking Soda

A dash of baking soda in coffee or tea will reduce acidity.

Sour Soups

The same applies to very sour soups. A pinch of baking soda will neutralize its acidity.

Baking Soda's Alkalinity Changes the Color of Foods

Baking soda is naturally alkaline. It raises the pH when added to liquids or foods.

The alkalinity of baking soda manifests by changing the color of some pigments in food. For example, sprinkling baking soda on purple cabbage or blueberries causes the anthocyanin in them to turn blue.

Use baking soda when baking green vegetables and they will have a bright green color.

Another fun experiment is to sprinkle baking soda on turmeric and watch the golden pigment of curcumin turn red.

Baking Soda as a Catalyst

Baking soda can also act as a catalyst in two important food reactions. A tiny pinch of baking soda added to foods while roasting or sautéing accelerates the rate of sugar caramelization, and supercharges the Maillard reaction. This is the rate at which the amino acids in proteins react with sugar, producing bittersweet, delicious flavor, a nut-like aroma, and gorgeous golden-brown hues.

The Double-Edged Sword of Baking Soda

After putting baking soda in our cakes and pies and muffins and breads to make them fluffy and tasty, which leads to possibly over-eating, the gastric discomfort can be calmed by ... baking soda!

Jekyll and Hyde Compound

Leavening requires an acidic catalyst in the batter, such as yogurt or buttermilk. When the acidic catalyst comes in contact with baking soda, in a simple acid-based reaction it causes the release of carbon dioxide.

But baking soda will also release smaller volumes of carbon dioxide *without* an acid by the process of "thermal decomposition," at temperatures above 50 degrees celsius (122 degrees Fahrenheit).

Thermal decomposition is dependent upon the temperature at which the substance chemically decomposes. Although this process is less preferred as it produces a bitter flavor.

Either way, whether the leavening is an added acidic catalyst, or dependent on heat only, the release of gas into the ingredients as they cook changes their density and texture.

Alchemy at its tastiest!

What is Baking Powder?

While baking soda is simply sodium bicarbonate, baking powder is composed of baking soda, which is slightly alkaline, and cream of tartar, a by-product of wine fermentation, which is slightly acidic. It's the clever invention of Eben Horsford.

These alkaline and acidic ingredients are kept from reacting by a buffer, each staying in their own corner, with a referee making sure that they do. This referee is usually cornstarch. Then, when they come in contact with liquid ingredients, the chemical reaction is stimulated.

Recipes That Call for Both Baking Soda and Baking Powder

That special tang in, for instance, buttermilk pancakes, requires both baking soda and baking powder. If only using baking soda, it will neutralize the acid of the but-termilk, and flatten the tangy flavor. The slightly acidic cream of tartar in the baking powder preserves the desired flavor.

On the other hand, baking soda helps the browning process of baked goods, and adding a bit of baking soda to a recipe that calls for baking powder only, can contribute to a beautifully brown baked product.

A Couple of Simple Tests

We take our baking soda and baking powder for granted, always patiently waiting for us in the cupboard, and may sometimes not recall how old they are. But these products *do* have a shelf life, and if it has been exceeded, you may be disappointed in the result of your lovely baking.

So here are a couple of simple tests to see if they are still viable:

Add a teaspoon of baking powder to a glass of hot water, and if it bubbles up, it's still active.

Add a teaspoon of vinegar to a teaspoon of baking soda in a glass, and, same thing, if it bubbles up, it's still good.

Be sure to transfer baking soda from the cardboard box to an airtight container, and store in a cool, dry place. You could also mark the date on the containers when you buy them.

Chapter High Points:

1. Baking soda is slightly alkaline with a pH between 8-9.5.

2. Baking soda is a leavening agent that makes baked goods rise.

3. A pinch of baking soda will improve the texture of baked vegetables, and reduce the gas-producing component of beans.

4. A dash of baking soda in bitter tea, coffee, or soups will reduce the bitter acidic flavor.

5. Baking powder is the addition of an acidic component to baking soda, usually cream of tartar, and a neutral component, usually cornstarch, to prevent chemical activation, until it is desired

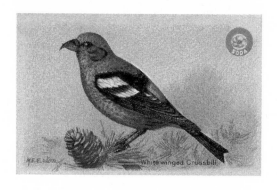

A Friend in Need

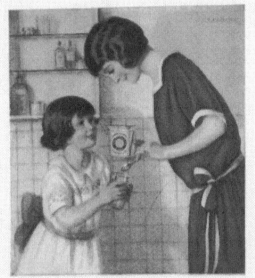

Facts worth knowing
about
BAKING SODA
as a proven medicinal agent

Chapter 4
Baking Soda and Health

B aking soda contains antimicrobial, anti-inflamma-tory, antiseptic, antifungal, antipruritic, and antibacterial properties!

WOW! Humble baking soda can help protect you from infections, discomforts, disorders, and diseases. Let's consider a few of them....

Baking Soda as an Anti-Fungal and Antibacterial

Baking soda kills various bacteria including streptococcus mutans, implicated in tooth decay. It is also effective against various fungal groups including yeasts, dermatophytes, and molds that cause skin and nail infections in humans and animals.

Baking Soda Treats Arthritis

One of the numerous ways that an overlay acidic body can let its discomfort be known is in the disease process of arthritis. Here, as with other diseases, toxins crystallize. Baking soda is outstanding in its ability to help remove this toxic acid and bring the body into pH balance. Through this process, the severity of arthritis symptoms is likely significantly reduced. If taken preventatively, it may even keep arthritis from manifesting altogether.

Baking Soda Balances pH

Baking soda's healing properties are primarily due to its being alkaline. Because of our diet, the environment, stress, EMFs, and so many other factors, we are bombarded with a pH imbalance. Baking soda can help to restore a healthy pH balance.

Baking Soda and the Bath

Be kind to your skin. It's our largest organ, and it's busy keeping out what needs to be kept out and holding in what needs to be held in. Taking a long, hot, soak in alkalizing baking soda is a defense for clearing away the toxins encountered on a daily basis, and preventing them from penetrating the skin.

Daily stresses take a toll on the body, as well as mind and spirit. Wash these stressors all away and relax, *truly relax*. Pour a cup of baking soda into the filling bath, and swish it around to make sure it's dissolved.

Sink into it, and become entirely present in the moment, filled with gratitude for this moment of peace and healing, while the neutralizing sodium bicarbonate removes oils, sweat, and acids from the skin, exfoliating imperfections and leaving your skin ultra soft and glowing.

Baking Soda Reduces Bloating and Gas

Mixing baking soda with water produces a bubbling reaction. Inside your body, this bubbling behavior can help release extra gas and the discomfort of bloating.

Baking Soda Treats Bronchitis

Inflammation of the bronchioles in the lungs leads to bronchitis. This inflammation can be reduced by drinking baking soda's alkaline water, relieving, and even potentially preventing, the symptoms of bronchitis.

Baking Soda a Bug Bite Soother

Make a paste with a teaspoon or two of baking soda and a few drops of water. Apply the soda paste on the bite repeatedly until it dissipates and stops itching.

Baking Soda in Cancer Research

As cancer is the second leading cause of death in the United States, there is considerable interest and research into approaches to healing.

With an acidic pH imbalance, unhealthy organisms in the body flourish, compromising the immune system, damaging organs and tissues, and developing various cancers. Baking soda increases the pH of acidic tumors, while not negatively affecting the pH of healthy tissues and blood.

Without an acidic environment, cancer is unable to survive. In addition, a balanced pH also gives nutritional and immune system support.

Oral doses of sodium bicarbonate have been shown in scientific research to inhibit spontaneous metastases in laboratory animals subjected to metastatic breast cancer, and to raise the tumor's pH.

Research is showing that baking soda helps chemotherapy work more effectively by making the tumor's environment less acidic.

Please observe the usual caveat to not embark on a baking soda regime without consulting your healthcare practitioner if you are healing from cancer.

Baking Soda Reduces Cold and Flu

People who consume baking soda regularly, scientific studies have shown, have reduced chances of getting colds or the flu, and they recover faster when they *do* get sick. Baking soda's ability to contribute to the body's pH balance is a significant factor in reducing colds and the flu.

Stir a quarter to half-a-teaspoon of baking soda, and half-a-teaspoon of salt in warm water, and gargle to alleviate a sore throat.

Then, slowly sip a warm glass of water with half-a-teaspoon of baking soda stirred into it, twice throughout the day.

Baking Soda – a Natural Deodorant

You can make a dusting of baking soda and cornstarch to apply to your underarms and feet. It will kill bacteria with its antibacterial property while absorbing moisture and sweat.

Baking Soda Helps Detox!

Baking soda water helps in the elimination of heavy metals and other toxic substances. Half-a-teaspoon in a glass of warm water on a daily basis goes a long way to help your body shed those toxins and heavy metals.

Baking Soda Calms Diarrhea and Upset Stomach

Stress, poor diet, certain medicines, and gastric reflux can trigger an upset stomach and diarrhea. Baking soda does double duty, treating digestive problems, and, again, contributing to the elimination of toxins.

Stir 1/2 teaspoon baking soda in a cup of warm water, and sip slowly. Do this up to three times a day. When you begin to feel better, reduce the baking soda intake.

Or add 1/2 teaspoon baking soda to a soothing, warm cup of peppermint tea.

Baking Soda for a Great Energy Boost!

Here's something to try. Drink half-a-teaspoon of baking soda in a glass of warm water before a workout to increase your energy.

During high-intensity exercise, muscle cells start to produce lactic acid, which is responsible for the burning sensation. Baking soda not only absorbs lactic acid, but also releases energy-providing hormones!

Studies have demonstrated that "bicarbonate loading" before exercise has a positive effect on athletic performance of sustained strenuous exercise, as well as being effective during prolonged physical activity involving intermittent high-intensity training. It reduces many of the negative side effects of high lactic acid in the muscles, with less damage and a more effective outcome. But, again, do not overdo it as excessive baking soda has potential negative side effects.

Baking soda helps delay fatigue due to its high pH, letting you perform at maximum intensity for longer. In one study, cyclists who drink a baking soda beverage before cycling, exercised an average of 4.5 minutes longer than those who didn't have any baking soda.

There is also support for drinking a glass of baking soda to reduce fatigue *post*-workout, or soaking in a tub of warm water with a half-cup of baking soda added to help neutralize lactic acid build-up in the muscles.

Baking Soda Removes Dark Circles Under the Eyes

Baking soda can brighten the skin under your eyes. Mix 2 teaspoons of baking soda with two teaspoons of chamomile tea. You can use water if you don't have tea. Stir the two ingredients into a paste and apply gently to the skin under your eyes.

Best practice is to lie back for fifteen to twenty minutes, totally relaxed, and let the alkaline process take effect. Consider it a mini meditation. Afterward, rinse off the baking soda and tea and admire your beautiful, radiant face.

Baking Soda Facial Exfoliation

Combine one or two tablespoons of baking soda with enough water to make a paste, and gently rub in a circular motion on your face to exfoliate your skin, then rinse. As the pH of healthy skin is slightly acidic, you do not want to over-alkalize it, so you may only want to do this once or twice a week. If you opt to exfoliate daily, be sure to follow with a quality moisturizer.

Baking Soda as a Foot Soother

Indulge your feet in a relaxing foot soak. In a small tub stir a couple tablespoons of baking soda in warm water. Then put your feet in, and sit back, with a long, contented sigh. R*elax!*

Not only will you shed a hard day, but the baking soda will remove sweat, odors, and bacteria, and even prevent toenail fungus. When you bring your feet out of the foot soak, give them a good, loving, massage, and maybe even add a bit of fragrant oil. Your feet work so hard for you every day. Give them some love!

Baking Soda Prevents or Helps Cure Gout

Excess uric acid in the blood can manifest as the extremely painful condition of gout. Uric acid crystallizes, and when it's crystallized, it cannot be flushed out of the body, unless and until it becomes more alkaline. Baking soda to the rescue! It is capable of alkalizing the internal environment, allowing the blood to flush out uric acid before it crystallizes.

Baking Soda as a Hand Cleanser and Softener

To neutralize odors on the hands, and exfoliate them and leave them super soft, prepare a paste with three parts baking soda and one part water, and scrub your hands. It will not only eliminate dirt but also any lingering odors, plus it acts as a gentle exfoliate, leaving hands soft and clean.

Baking Soda for Super Clean Hair

Add a teaspoon or two of baking soda to shampoo in the palm of your hand, and apply to hair and scalp. It will remove hairdressing products and all the residues from a busy life, leaving your hair beautifully clean, soft, and manageable.

Baking Soda Removes Dandruff

Get rid of itchy dandruff, which is, of course, acidic. The scalp is not in its best PH balance, but this can be solved with the application of baking soda. Pour one to two tablespoons of dry baking soda into your palm, then apply to your wet scalp and hair. Let it soak for a minute or two, then rinse out.

Follow this routine on a weekly basis, and dandruff will be banished!

Baking Soda – Brush and Comb Cleaner

Combine two tablespoons of baking soda with half-cup of water, making a paste. Coat brushes and combs, then let them sit for a while. Rinse thoroughly.

Baking Soda for Heartburn and Indigestion Relief

Heartburn can occur for a variety of reasons, among them eating large meals, eating greasy, spicy foods, and/or drinking carbonated beverages, overdoing alcohol, etc. Heartburn, or acid reflux, is caused by the stomach's acids moving up into the esophagus.

Baking soda effectively reduces the pain and discomfort of heartburn and indigestion. Add half-a-teaspoon of baking soda to a cup of warm water and sip until gone. Do not overdo as it is possible to become overly alkaline.

Another thing to keep in mind is that baking soda is very high in sodium, an important factor if limiting sodium intake.

Baking Soda Can Treat Hyperkalemia

Hyperkalemia is a serious condition, and you must co-ordinate any baking soda protocol with your healthcare provider. Hyperkalemia is when there are dangerously high potassium levels in the blood, above 6.0 millimoles per liter.

Common causes of hyperkalemia are kidney diseases, diabetes, dehydration, an injury, or excessive use of potassium supplements and beta-blockers.

As most people have a potassium *insufficiency*, a high potassium level is cause for concern. Baking soda is a possible temporary remedy if hyperkalemia is caused by acidosis, as it will contribute to neutralizing overly acidic blood. Your healthcare provider may recommend half-a-teaspoon of baking soda on a daily basis in a glass of warm water.

Baking Soda Treats Infections

Baking soda, both internally and topically, is quite effective for quick recovery from infections. As a natural antiseptic, topically, it can treat and disinfect wounds.

As a drink, baking soda dissolved in a glass of water attends to internal infections, preventing further infections, both inside and out!

Baking Soda Reduces Inflammation

Along this same vein, much inflammation is caused by a pH imbalance, resulting in an acidic environment. A half-a-teaspoon of baking soda stirred into a glass of warm water, and sipped slowly, can help reduce the acidic inflammation.

Baking Soda for Itchy Skin Relief

Itchy skin rashes are irritating but common problems, whether from allergic rashes, sunburn, or plant materials such as poison ivy or poison oak. Since baking soda is antiseptic and anti-inflammatory, applying it topically is soothing and healing, alleviating itching, swelling, and inflammation.

Add three parts baking soda to one part water to make a paste. Apply the paste to the affected area, and let it dry. Repeat this procedure as necessary until the irritation has resolved.

Conversely, as I oft repeat, a nice long soak in a baking soda bath can be quite healing. Add one cup of baking soda to a warm bathtub of water and soak for at least fifteen minutes.

Afterward, mix some baking soda in with your body lotion, which will additionally calm itchiness.

Baking Soda Helps Keep Kidneys Healthy

Kidneys are vital because they remove excess waste, toxins, and water from the blood while balancing important minerals like potassium, sodium, and calcium, and promoting healthy hormone production.

Baking soda's alkalinity buffers bodily acids, while keeping pH levels balanced. Because low-functioning kidneys have a hard time removing acid from the body, consuming baking soda can help those processes. Research has shown that baking soda even slows the progress of chronic kidney disease.

For example, studies conducted at the Royal Hospital in London have shown that baking soda has a positive effect on kidney function and slows the formation of kidney stones.

In addition, it has helped people on dialysis. A study that lasted two years, included patients on dialysis who were daily given baking soda. At the end of the study, the results were absolutely astonishing: only six-and-a-half percent of the patients consuming baking soda still needed dialysis!

A daily cup of baking soda water can help regulate the body's pH, and improve its hormone balance, nutrient absorption, and the quality of the blood—all of which help keep the kidneys healthy.

Baking Soda Boosts Kidney Health

One-hundred-and-thirty-four patients with chronic kidney disease (CKD) and low blood bicarbonate levels were the subjects of a clinical study published in the *Journal of the American Society of Nephrology*.

The participants who supplemented with baking soda on a daily basis experienced a significant slowing in the progression of their kidney disease. Even more impressively, fewer patients in the baking soda group developed end-stage renal disease (ESRD) compared to those in the control group.

Baking Soda Can Decrease and Prevent Kidney Stone Formation

Kidney stones are formed by an ionic imbalance in the body, which causes urine to become too acidic. The acidic, concentrated minerals frequently crystallize and stick together, forming kidney stones. Passing kidney stones is quite painful, with pain radiating to the lower abdomen and groin.

Baking soda contributes to balancing both the pH and the ions, leading to less acidic crystallization staying *in* the body, and more waste *exiting* the body, thus preventing the formation of kidney stones, and helping to dissolve existing ones.

A suggested dosage in the medical literature is—no surprises here—to mix half-a-teaspoon baking soda in a glass of warm water to help dissolve kidney stones. Drink this mixture twice a day.

⚠ CAUTION: *Please heed my oft-repeated caution to not overdo baking soda intake, especially in regard to the kidneys. Which, although it can be healing, it can also trigger metabolic acidosis. As always, orchestrate this protocol with your trusted healthcare practitioner.*

Baking Soda Reduces LDL Cholesterol

Baking soda's alkaline pH helps with the reduction and prevention of LDL (low-density lipids) cholesterol. Drink half-a-teaspoon of baking soda a day dissolved in a glass of warm water.

Baking Soda as a Mouthwash and Whitening Toothpaste

Baking soda is often found in toothpaste due to its ability to remove dental plaque. But you can use baking soda by itself as a perfectly good tooth cleaner.

Make a paste by adding a couple of drops of water to half a teaspoon of baking soda, or simply dip your brush in a small container of baking soda at your bathroom sink, specifically for this purpose.

Along with keeping your teeth healthy and clean and neutralizing acidic bacteria in the mouth, you will also notice that baking soda whitens teeth over time. Stains will disappear. Do keep in mind that baking soda is slightly abrasive and you will want to brush gently so as not to damage tooth enamel.

Also, a baking soda mouthwash freshens your breath with its antibacterial and antimicrobial properties, increasing the pH level of the mouth, significantly inhibiting bacterial growth.

To make a baking soda mouthwash, add half-a-teaspoon of baking soda to half-a-glass of warm water.

Baking Soda Soothes and Heals Canker Sores

Canker sores are painful ulcers inside the mouth. A baking soda mouthwash, as noted above, will soothe the pain, and speed up the healing process of canker sores. You can also place a small amount of baking soda powder on the sore a couple times a day.

Baking Soda Treats Nail Fungus

A nail fungus can cause your nail to discolor, crumble along the edge, and/or thicken. It usually starts as a white spot under the tip of the nail. Soak it in baking soda and water.

Or make a paste of a couple teaspoons of baking soda and water, and apply it to the nail, leaving it on as long as you comfortably can. Do this once or twice a day until the infection heals.

Another option is to mix two tablespoons of baking soda with half-cup of apple cider vinegar. Dip your nails in this solution for five minutes, twice a day.

Baking Soda Applied to Pimples and Acne

Because of baking soda's antiseptic and anti-inflammatory properties, it can reduce the symptoms of acne by balancing the skin's pH.

Mix two parts of baking soda to one part water to make a paste. Apply to the acne and let it sit two to five minutes, then thoroughly wash it off. Repeat this process for three days, then only once or twice per week because, although acne is a problem with acidic skin, the goal is to have a pH balance, and not end up with skin that is too alkaline.

Baking Soda Helps to Quit Smoking

Smoking is extremely acidic. Alkalizing baking powder has been effective for many people to help them with their desire to quit smoking.

There are two possible methods that have been observed as effective. One is to put a teaspoon of baking soda in a glass of warm water, stir until it dissolves, and sip it.

The other method is simply to touch a few granules of dry baking soda to the tongue which will immediately alkalize your mouth, and if you really mean to "kick the habit," there will be a natural revulsion against the extremely acidic input of a cigarette and its smoke.

This commitment must also be accompanied by a healthy alkaline diet, meaningful exercise, and restful sleep. Orchestrate these components to attain your excellent life!

Freshen your breath! Brighten your world!

Baking Soda – Amazing Splinter Remover

Splinters or slivers can be very painful and annoying. But, surprisingly, a paste of two parts baking soda to one part water applied to the splinter and bandaged will cause the sliver to back out in a day or two, so that it can be readily removed. Try it!

Baking Soda Eases Ulcer Pain

Although baking powder cannot cure your ulcer, it can reduce the pain. Ulcers are caused by a reduction of the mucus that protects the stomach from its own digestive juices. Alkaline baking soda can provide temporary protection.

Baking Soda and Urinary Tract Infections

Urinary tract infections (UTIs) are the number one infection people get and are more common in women. They are very painful and bring the daily routine to a halt. A UTI is treated with antibiotics, but as antibiotics become less effective the more they are used, it's better to keep the system in good health.

Because baking soda is antiseptic and alkaline, drinking baking soda water helps clean and heal the urinary system, including the blood, the urinary tract, and the bladder, hopefully maintaining the system in a healthy condition so that antibiotics are not required.

The effects of baking soda is the subject of a study with a group of thirty-three women who had urinary tract infections, and acidic urine with a pH below six. After drinking baking soda dissolved in water for four weeks, their urine became properly pH balanced, with an accompanying significant level of positive effects on symptoms.

Baking Soda During a Medical Crisis

Doctors use a five percent sodium bicarbonate infusion in medical crises such as severe renal failure, a heart attack, uncontrolled diabetes, and other critical situations.

Chapter High Points:

1. The chapter opened with this amazing statement, and it's worth repeating: baking soda contains antimicrobial, anti-inflammatory, antiseptic, antifungal, antipruritic, and antibacterial properties.

2. Baking soda attacks the various toxins that crystallize in the body, and see to it that they get removed, bringing the body into harmonious pH balance.

3. Baking soda neutralizes many different bacteria. Its power over bacteria is an ongoing discovery for scientists the world around.

4. We can't ask for a better security guard. Baking soda never tires of checking the perimeter, working to keep out of the body what is harmful, and keep in what is healthful—despite our own frequent, unwise choices.

5. Baking soda contributes to a healthy circadian rhythm. *Sleep tight!*

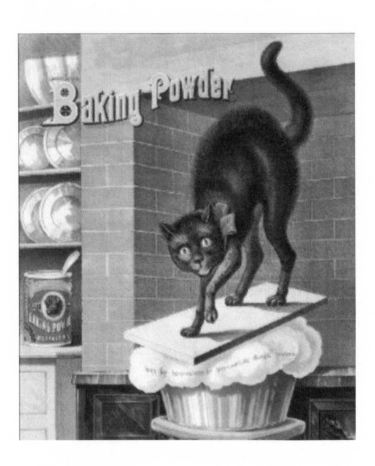

Chapter 5
Baking Soda and Household Uses

There are so many uses for alkaline baking soda, a great cleaner and deodorizer! Following is a list, which is by no means exhaustive, of the many ways affordable, effective baking soda can be used around the home, the car, and the yard.

Can you think of other ways to use baking soda, not on this list?

Baking Soda as an Air Freshener

Baking soda is an excellent and much healthier alternative to commercial air fresheners, as it neutralizes odor rather than masks it, and, perhaps even more important, it is free of industrial chemicals.

Pour half-cup of baking soda into a small jar.

Add fifteen to twenty drops of your favorite aromatic essential oil.

Cover the jar with a bit of colorful cloth that matches the decor, and tie a string or ribbon around the fabric.

All you need to do is occasionally give the jar a shake to stir up the lovely aroma.

Baking Soda–Multipurpose Bathroom Cleaner

You can't beat baking soda for a cleaner in the bathroom! Commercial cleaners are expensive. Baking soda's antibacterial component disinfects as it cleans, and brightens the many bathroom surfaces.

Make a paste of three parts baking soda to one part water and apply to the surfaces to be cleaned. Let it sit for twenty minutes, then wipe it down with a damp cloth or sponge.

Baking Soda – Carpet Cleaner

Carpet cleaners are made of chemicals that are potentially harmful to pets and children, or even, for that matter, adults! Use baking soda for a good cleaning and odor removal for your carpet.

Sprinkle baking soda on the carpet and let it sit over night. It absorbs orders and alkalizes the carpet.

Then vacuum up the baking soda. Your vacuum cleaner will be full of baking soda and need to be emptied. By the way, the vacuum cleaner will be odor neutralized and alkalized too!

Carpet Stain Remover

Baking soda and vinegar together make a compound called carbonic acid, which is a common ingredient in many cleaning products. The two together have a fizzing reaction, which contributes to breaking down tough stains.

First, sprinkle a layer of baking soda over the carpet stain.

Fill a spray bottle with equal amounts of vinegar and water, and spray over the baking soda.

Allow it to thoroughly dry, then scrub the baking soda loose with a brush, and vacuum.

Surprise! The stain is gone!

Baking Soda – Closet Freshener

To freshen your closet, place a box or cup of baking soda inside. Occasionally replace with new baking soda in order to keep the closet smelling fresh.

Baking Soda – Coffee and Teapot Cleaner

To remove coffee stains and unpleasant tastes from the coffee or teapot, mix one-fourth-cup of baking soda with one quart of warm water. Rub the mixture on and in the pots to clean. If encountering a tough stain, let it sit overnight, then finish washing in the morning and rinse.

Baking Soda Deodorizes the Cutting Board

Sprinkle the kitchen cutting board with baking soda. Scrub and rinse to remove not only odors but also any and all lingering bacteria.

Baking Soda in the Dishwasher

Baking soda helps to remove food debris and grease from dishes and pots and pans. Add two tablespoons of baking soda to the regular dishwashing detergent.

Baking Soda Unclogs Drains

You will need boiling water and vinegar in addition to baking soda to unclog a drain.

Fill a large pot with water and bring it to a boil, then pour it down the drain.

Follow with half-cup of baking soda and let it sit for five to ten minutes.

Then make a pint mixture of a cup of vinegar in a cup of very hot water, and pour it down the drain.

Let it sit for another ten minutes, followed by more boiling water. Now you have an unclogged drain that has bacteria flushed away and is smelling fresh!

Baking Soda for Fabrics

Increase the Power of Laundry Detergent

Refresh the laundry with one-half-cup of alkaline baking soda added to the washing machine's rinse cycle, leaving the laundry cleaner and brighter, and the whites whiter. It also reduces static electricity.

For stubborn stains, add one-half-cup of baking soda to the liquid detergent on the wash cycle, to boost the detergent's action. It will also soften the water, and you may need less detergent.

Cleaning Cloth Diapers

Baking soda can be helpful in cleaning baby's cloth diapers. Dissolve half-cup of baking soda in two quarts of water and soak the diapers, then rinse.

Remove Odors from Stuffed Animals

Sprinkle stuffed toys with a baking soda dry shower to keep them smelling fresh. Let the baking soda sit for fifteen minutes (or longer). Then remove the baking soda with a brush or gentle vacuuming.

Baking Soda Will Put out the Fire!

A minor grease fire in the kitchen can be extinguished with baking soda. Baking soda on a fire causes it to produce carbon dioxide, which stifles the flames.

Baking Soda as a Floor Cleaner

Baking soda removes dirt and grime from non-waxed floors and tiles. Use one-half cup of baking soda in a bucket of warm water. For scuff marks, gently scrub the mark with powdered baking soda and a clean damp sponge, then rinse.

Baking Soda – Fridge Odor Neutralizer

Baking soda freshens a smelly fridge by neutralizing bad odors. It actually neutralizes the odor particles, rather than just masking the smell. The smells can come from strong acids, for example, spoiled milk, or from strong alkaline, for example, rotten fish. Baking soda shifts both acidic and alkaline unpleasant orders to a neutral odorless state.

An open box of baking soda in the back of the fridge will have this neutralizing effect on odors.

Baking Soda – Fruit and Veggie Scrub

Baking soda is a safe way to clean dirt, debris, and acidic pesticides from fresh fruits and vegetables. Sprinkle baking soda on a damp, clean sponge, then gently scrub the fruit or veggie, and rinse.

Or you could leave the fruits and vegetables to soak in the sink for a while in water and a-quarter-cup to half-cup of baking soda.

Baking Soda Cleans Furniture

Baking soda will clean and remove all sorts of marks, including crayons, from painted walls and furniture. Apply it to a damp sponge and rub on the marking lightly, then wipe clean afterward with a clean, dry cloth.

Baking Soda as a Kitchen Cleaner

Baking soda makes a great kitchen cleaner!

When used in paste form or dry on a damp sponge, its crystalline structure provides a gentle abrasion that removes tough dirt without scratching the surface, and its alkalinity cuts through acidic fats contained in dirt and grease, then is dissolved in a water rinse to sparkling clean!

Add a few drops of your favorite essential oil to add a pleasant, natural fragrance to your environment.

Baking Soda Cleans the Microwave

Baking soda applied to a clean damp sponge will clean the microwave in just a few moments. After it's spanking clean, rinse it down with water.

Baking Soda Cleans the Oven

Why not avoid the harmful chemicals that oven cleaners are generally made of? It's easier and less expensive and healthier to use baking soda.

Sprinkle baking soda on the bottom of the oven, then spray with water and let stand overnight. In the morning, rub and remove the baking soda and dirt with a sponge.

Baking Soda and Paint and Corrosion Removal

Baking soda is used in a process known as soda blasting to remove corrosion, more gently than the usual sand product used for blasting.

Baking Soda – Pots and Pans Cleaner

Let pots and pans soak for twenty minutes in the sink in a baking soda solution of a cup of baking soda to the sink filled to cover the pots and pans in hot water. They will clean right up with just a bit of elbow grease, alkaline fresh!

A scorched pot can be a real challenge to clean. Cover the bottom of the pot with baking soda and add just enough water to cover the burnt areas. Bring it to a boil, then empty the pan. If stains still remain, give it a bit of attention with the scouring pad and gently remove the remaining stain.

Baking Soda – Recyclables and Garbage Odor Eliminator

Sprinkle baking soda on the bottom of trash cans to keep them odor-free. It helps eliminate garbage smells by literally neutralizing the bad odor molecules.

Sprinkle baking soda on the top of the recyclables container for the same effect.

In addition, occasionally clean the trash cans and recyclable containers by sprinkling baking soda on a damp sponge, scrub them down and rinse.

Baking Soda for Septic Care

Use baking soda in the drains on a regular basis to help the septic system flow freely. One cup of baking soda per week poured down the drain will help maintain an alkaline pH in your septic tank.

Baking Soda – Shoe Deodorizer

Baking soda is great for deodorizing your shoes. Sprinkle it inside the shoes, and the odor will clear up within minutes.

Baking Soda – Shower Curtain Cleaner

Rub baking soda on shower curtain stains, then turn on the shower and the stains will go down the drain.

Baking Soda as a Silverware Polish – Easy Peasy Method

Make a paste that is three parts baking soda and one part water. Rub it on the silverware and let it sit in a large tray. After fifteen to twenty minutes, rinse the silverware. It's now all shiny and silver.

Baking Soda as a Silverware Polish – Big Guns Method

Here's a baking soda silverware cleaning method for silver that is heavily tarnished.

In a baking pan that is lined with aliminum foil add the following:

1 tablespoon baking soda
1/2 cup white vinegar
1 cup boiling water

Then place the silver in the pan. The tarnish will begin to disappear immediately. As soon as the silver looks shiny, you can remove it. Heavily tarnished silverware may need to sit in the mixture longer.

The silver is undergoing a chemical reaction with the aluminum foil, baking soda, and vinegar. The tarnish is transferred from the silverware onto the aluminum pan. It may leave a pale yellow residue in the pan.

Baking Soda Cleans Stainless Steel, Pewter, and Copper

All these metals become bright, shiny, and new with a good baking soda paste session. You can clean your jewelry, pocket change, and Tupperware with baking soda, too!

Baking Soda Removes Odors from Sponges

Soak sponges in a solution of one-quarter-cup of baking powder to a quart of water to clean and remove odors.

Baking Soda Cleans Sports Equipment

Use a solution of four tablespoons of baking soda to one quart of warm water to clean and deodorize sports equipment.

Sprinkle baking soda on golf bags and sports bags to deodorize them.

Baking Soda for Washing the Car

Baking soda readily removes grease, dirt, tree sap, insects, tar, bad smells, etc., and is the perfect product to clean and refresh your car. Make a paste of three tablespoons of baking soda and one cup of warm water.

Rub this paste onto tires, lights, seats, windows, chrome, floor mats—everything but the paint, and then rinse.

For the paint finish, add a half-cup of baking soda to a gallon of water, stirring until it is thoroughly dissolved. Baking soda is a good alkaline cleaner, but in its powdered state, it *is* abrasive. Apply with a soft sponge, and rinse. Now your car is all bright and shiny!

In between washing, odors can be eliminated by sprinkling dry, powdered, baking soda on fabric seats and carpets. Let it sit for a while to absorb the odors, and then vacuum it up.

Baking Soda Removes Grease Stains From Garage Floor

Baking soda is perfect for cleaning oil and grease that inevitably make their way to the garage floor. Sprinkle baking soda on the spot and rub with a wet brush.

Baking Soda to Clean Car Batteries

Baking soda will neutralize corrosive battery acid in cars, mowers, tractors, etc., because it is a mild alkaline. Be sure to disconnect the battery terminals before cleaning.

Use a paste of three parts baking soda to one part water, and scrub the corrosion off the battery terminals. Applying petroleum jelly to the terminals after cleaning will help prevent further corrosion.

Love Your Pets!

Baking Soda as a Kitty-Litter Deodorizer

Baking soda is useful for pets too! Naturally deodorize your kitty's box by sprinkling the bottom of the box with baking soda, then adding the kitty litter.

Baking Soda to Deodorize Pet Beds

Remove odors from pet beds by sprinkling them with baking soda. Wait fifteen minutes or even overnight for stronger odors, then vacuum.

Baking Soda to Dry Shampoo Your Cat or Dog

Baking soda also works as an odor eliminator for pets. First, brush your cat or dog, then rub baking soda into the fur and massage it into their skin, avoiding their eyes.

Leave the baking soda for five minutes, and then brush it out of the fur. Finish by rubbing the fur down with a dry towel to be sure to remove the baking soda. A little bit of baking soda is harmless for a pet to ingest, but it should be kept at a minimum.

Consult your vet before using baking soda if you have concerns that your pet might be allergic to it if your pet tends to have allergies.

Baking Soda to Get Rid of Skunk Smell

If your pet—or even you!—encounters a skunk, here is a recipe to deal with the odor. Add one-quarter-cup baking soda to a quart of three percent hydrogen peroxide and rub down the area of offending odor.

Baking Soda - A Homemade Weed Killer

Baking soda makes an effective weed killer. It's high in sodium, which plants do not like.

Sprinkle baking soda over weeds in areas that they do not share with your garden plants or flowers, because it will damage those plants as well.

Baking Soda for Pest Control

Baking soda mixed with a bit of sugar strategically placed on their path will eradicate insects like cockroaches, ants, and others.

Baking Soda As a Cattle Feed Supplement

Baking soda is a natural feed additive used to improve the health and performance of cows. It is a good source of B vitamins, minerals, and fiber.

Creative Ideas with Baking Soda

Baking Soda and Super Glue

Baking soda and superglue have a special relationship. Baking soda builds up with superglue and becomes *super strong*. You can repair miscellaneous broken items with this method.

Carefully put a dab of superglue on the broken part and then put a little baking soda on the superglue. Continue this process, back and forth, as you fill in a crack, or build up the structure of a broken piece. You might want to practice this a bit before working with the actual item.

You may also need to get inventive if the part or repair is very small or hard to get at. Toothpicks, tiny screwdrivers, or other "tools" may need to be devised. Be careful to not make yourself a part of the repair! The created part or repair can be sanded with a fingernail file.

With practice, you may discover that you're able to put new life into a slew of broken items!

Air-Dry Clay with Baking Soda

Why spend a lot of money on expensive air dry clay, when you can make your own, and color it just exactly the color you want? Here's a simple recipe. Have fun making sculptures:

Half-cup of cornstarch

1 cup of baking soda

Three-quarter cup of cold water

Stir these three ingredients together, then put on the stove on medium heat, and stir until it's like mashed potatoes

Remove from the heat and place the clay on a plate

Cover with a damp paper towel until it cools

Use food coloring to make your clay any color you want And now, let your imagination run wild creating fun and interesting sculptures!

Add Baking Soda to Latex or Acrylic Paint

Adding baking soda to latex or acrylic paint will give it structure so that when you paint it or otherwise get creative with how you apply it, it has depth and texture.

Add a quarter-cup to a half-cup of baking soda to a quart of paint and stir thoroughly. You'll see that it's rather "fluffy." You may need to experiment with how much baking soda you want in the paint, depending on the effect you're going for.

Happy creating!

Chapter High Points:

1. Baking soda works inside and outside of the home to keep it in pH balance.

2. Odors, dirt, grease, oil, and stains are all banished with the application of baking soda, whether applied as a dry powder, a liquid with baking soda stirred into water or vinegar, or a paste.

3. Baking soda is as helpful and healthful to our pets and livestock as to us.

4. Acids of all kinds, in our clothes, in the refrigerator, in the drain, on the garage floor, etc., are neutralized by sodium bicarbonate's slight but effective alkalinity.

5. Do you love to have things shiny and clean? So does baking soda! Its mild abrasive quality works wonders on so many surfaces, from spoons to the car's wheels and everything in between.

Good Things to Eat

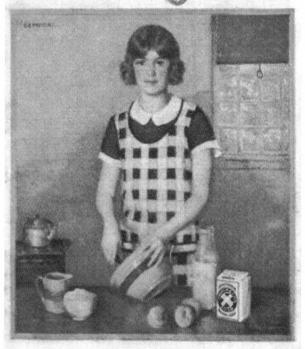

MADE WITH

BAKING SODA

Chapter 6
Yummy Tummy Baking Soda Baked Goodies

L et's put into practical use all of this contemplation of baking soda and its preferred occupation of making heart-warming, happy-tummy, baked goods ... with a few delicious recipes!

Pecan Snickerdoodles

Ingredients:

2-1/2 cups flour

1 cup finely chopped pecans

2 tsp. cream of tartar

3 tsp. baking soda

2 Tbsp apple cider vinegar

1/2 tsp. salt

1 cup butter or margarine, softened

1 3/4 cups sugar, divided

1 tsp. ground cinnamon

Instructions:

Heat oven to 375°F.

Mix first 5 ingredients in large bowl

Beat butter and 1-1/2 cups sugar in large bowl with mixer until light and fluffy

Gradually beat in flour mixture until well-blended

Shape into 1-inch balls

Mix remaining sugar and cinnamon

Roll balls in cinnamon sugar

Place on baking sheets

Bake 10 to 12 minutes or until lightly browned

Cool on baking sheets for a couple minutes

Remove to wire racks to cool completely.

Then watch them disappear!

Pumpkin Muffins

How to make almond meal follows the banana bread instructions, below. Almond meal is great to add to lots of recipes, or sprinkle on hot cereal or even in your salad. Lots of nutrition with a light touch of marzipan flavor!

Ingredients:

2 Tbsp mashed ripe banana

3/4 cup pumpkin puree

2/3 cup brown sugar

1/4 cup maple syrup

1/4 cup olive oil

1 tsp vanilla extract

3 tsp baking soda

1/4 tsp sea salt

1/2 tsp ground cinnamon

1 1/4 tsp pumpkin pie spice

1/2 cup water

2 Tbsp vinegar

1/2 cup almond meal (recipe below)

3/4 cup rolled oats or gluten-free rolled oats

1 cup flour

Topping:

3 Tbsp brown sugar

3 1/2 Tbsp flour

2 Tbsp chopped pecans or walnuts

1 1/4 Tbsp coconut oil

pinch of cinnamon

pinch of pumpkin pie spice

Instructions:

Preheat oven to 350 degrees F (174 C)

Lightly grease the muffin tins and dust with flour, or line with paper liners

Mash the banana in a bowl

Add pumpkin purée, maple syrup, brown sugar, olive oil, and vanilla extract and stir until combined

Stir in baking soda, salt, cinnamon, and pumpkin pie spice

Add water and vinegar, stir

Add almond meal, oats, and flour and stir until just combined

Fill the muffin tins

Topping:

In a bowl, add brown sugar, flour, nuts, coconut oil, cinnamon, and pumpkin pie spice

Mash ingredients together with a fork

Top muffins with this topping

Bake for 30 minutes or until they are golden brown and a toothpick comes out clean

Let cool for 5 minutes in the muffin tin, then remove and cool on a cooling rack.

Perfect for an afternoon tea!

Blackberry Cornmeal Muffins

Ingredients:

1/4 cup dairy or dairy-free milk

2 Tbsp apple cider vinegar

3 tsp baking soda

2 Tbsp maple syrup

1/2 cup cane sugar

1/4 cup melted butter or oil

3/4 cup unsweetened applesauce

1/4 tsp sea salt

1/4 cup almond meal

1 cup fine cornmeal

1 cup unbleached all-purpose flour

1 cup blackberries – cut into large pieces and tossed in flour

Instructions:

Preheat oven to 350 degrees F (176 C)

Line a muffin tin with paper liners, or lightly grease the tins and coat with flour

In a bowl add milk, apple cider vinegar, and baking soda

Stir ingredients and set aside

In another bowl, add maple syrup, sugar, and melted butter or oil

Stir vigorously until sugar is dissolved

Add applesauce and salt and stir to combine. Then add almond milk mixture and stir

Add almond meal, cornmeal, and flour and stir until just combined

The batter will be thick

Gently fold the blackberries into the batter

Scoop batter into muffin tins until they're almost full

Bake for 25-30 minutes, until a toothpick comes out clean

Let cool for 15-20 minutes in the pan, then lift out. Let cool completely on a cooling rack

Delish!!

Super-Duper Chocolate Cake

Ingredients:
2 cups milk or dairy-free alternative
1 Tbsp apple cider vinegar
2/3 cup coconut oil, melted
2 tsp pure vanilla extract
1 1/4 cups unsweetened applesauce
2 1/4 cups flour or gluten-free flour
1 1/3 cups sugar
1 cup unsweetened cocoa powder
2 tsp baking soda
1 tsp baking powder
1/4 tsp salt

Frosting:

1 cup butter or margarine

2 1/2 – 3 cups powdered sugar

2/3 cup unsweetened cocoa powder

1/4 cup semisweet chocolate (melted and slightly cooled)

2 tsp pure vanilla extract

~1/4 cup milk or dairy free alternative

Instructions:

Preheat oven to 350 degrees F (176 C)

Lightly spray two 8-inch round cake pans or one sheet pan with nonstick spray and dust with cocoa powder

Mix the milk and vinegar in a large mixing bowl, and let set for a few minutes to activate

Add the oil, vanilla extract, and applesauce and beat until foamy.

If coconut oil hardens, microwave for 10-15 seconds or until melted

Add the flour, sugar, cocoa powder, baking soda, baking powder, and salt to a sifter and slowly sift over the wet ingredients while mixing with a hand-held or standing mixer

Mix until it is creamy

Pour batter into the pans

Bake 30-40 minutes, until a toothpick inserted into the center comes out clean

Let cool completely before frosting

Buttercream Frosting:

Prepare frosting by beating together the butter or margarine, powdered sugar, cocoa powder, semisweet chocolate (melted and slightly cooled), vanilla extract, and milk until light and fluffy.

Add the powdered sugar in small amounts, then beat.

Frost the cake generously after it has cooled.

Happy unbirthday!

Almond Banana Bread

Fun, super-tasty banana bread, made with *almond meal.*

Ingredients:
3 medium ripe bananas (~1 1/2 cups)
1/2 tsp pure vanilla extract
3 Tbsp coconut oil, melted
1/4 cup cane sugar
1/4 cup packed brown sugar
2-3 Tbsp maple syrup
4 tsp baking powder
1 Tbsp apple vinegar
3/4 tsp sea salt
1/2 tsp ground cinnamon
3/4 cup dairy or non-dairy milk
1 1/4 cup almond meal

1 1/4 cup flour or gluten-free flour

1 1/4 cup oats or gluten-free oats

Instructions:

Preheat oven to 350 degrees F (176 C) and line a 9×5-inch loaf pan with parchment paper

Mash banana in a large bowl. Add vanilla, oil, cane sugar, brown sugar, maple syrup, baking powder, vinegar, salt, cinnamon, milk or non-dairy milk, and beat vigorously

Then add the almond meal, flour, and oats and stir until combined

Bake for 1 hour 10 minutes. Test its readiness—it should feel firm and be golden brown.

Let cool completely to firm up before cutting.

Almond Meal

Ingredient:

1 1/2 cups raw, sliced, or whole, almonds

Instructions:

Add almonds to blender. Turn the blender on the highest setting for 5-10 seconds, then stop and scrape and stir the nuts to blend clumps, and repeat this process until the nuts become powdery. Don't blend too long or the nuts will turn into almond butter.

Chocolate Chip Cookies

Ingredients:

1/2 cup butter or dairy-free butter

1/4 cup granulated sugar

1/2 cup packed brown sugar

1 1/2 cups flour

1 teaspoon baking soda

1 teaspoon vanilla

1-3 tablespoons water

2 tablespoons vegetable oil

1 cup chocolate chips, or more

1/2 cup walnuts, or your favorite nut, and more if you want 'em!

Instructions:

Preheat the oven to 350F

Put butter and sugars in a bowl and mix 1-2 minutes with a mixer, until creamy

Mix in flour and baking soda

Then add water, oil, and vanilla and mix together. Batter should hold together nicely, neither sticky nor crumbly – the variation in water is what comes into play. Environment and altitude can have an effect on the batter

Fold in the chocolate chips and nuts

Drop by spoonful onto ungreased baking sheet. Make the cookies the size you like, but keep in mind that smaller cookies bake faster, and larger cookies need more oven time. With that in mind bake for 9 to 12 minutes.

Everybody's favorite! And the kitchen smells lovely!

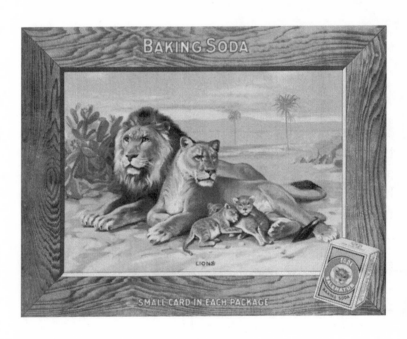

BAKING SODA

LIONS

SMALL CARD IN EACH PACKAGE

Chapter 7
Exciting Science – Baking Soda and Research

A team of research scientists conducted experiments showing that bicarbonate enhanced the activity of some antibiotics. In regard to sepsis, bicarbonate increased the impact of antibiotics on four of the bacterial species identified by the World Health Organization as global health concerns.

They hypothesized that bicarbonate interferes with the energy available to bacteria by altering the proton motive force (PMF). This is an electrochemical force across the bacterial cell wall that bacteria harness to make energy. Bicarbonate interferes with this force, which can, in turn, influence how the antibiotic molecules behave.

For instance, the proton motive force is hooked up to pumps that bacteria possess within their cell membranes. Measuring bacteria's degree of sensitivity to antibiotics is expressed as "minimum inhibitory concentrations" (MIC). That is to say, the concentration of antibiotic necessary to stop bacterial growth.

The researchers posed the question, "Does bicarbonate, by itself, have antimicrobial effects?" While sodium bicarbonate is reducing the pH gradient, bacteria is busily compensating by increasing the electrical gradient.

Aminoglycosides are a group of broad-spectrum antibiotics with activity that is related to electrical charge. Bicarbonate enhances the entry of aminoglycosides, which are thought to work by inhibiting protein synthesis inside bacteria. In simplest terms, kill rates of bacteria are increased when higher concentrations of aminoglycosides are present.

Can Baking Soda Fight Sepsis?

Sepsis interferes with the efficient use of oxygen by cells, that switch to pathways that produce less energy and a build-up of metabolic acids, which lower the pH.

The body holds on to alkaline bicarbonate and increases the respiratory rate to blow off carbon dioxide, an acid. But as sepsis intensifies, the kidneys cannot hold on to enough bicarbonate, and the respiratory rate cannot go fast enough to compensate. The individual's pH becomes more acidic.

Oxygen binds more tightly to hemoglobin in an acidic environment, while less and less is released to the tissue that needs it for energy production, resulting in more metabolic acids and a continued lowering of pH.

The other consequence of the increasingly inefficient energy utilization is that the heart begins to fail. To maintain adequate flow, blood vessels dilate so that the heart does not have to work as hard. Physicians administer drugs to increase the pumping ability of the heart and adjust the blood vessels to optimize circulation. But, as these drugs are less effective in acidic environments, physicians provide supplemental bicarbonate to improve the drug's action and support the pumping of the heart.

The current clinical belief is that the role of bicarbonate is to support circulation. But it is now theorized that bicarbonate has a greater role than merely supporting circulation and that it's possible to improve the outcome of sepsis by supporting the body's stores of bicarbonate earlier. Bicarbonate may prove to be a simple means to improve care for seriously ill people, with an inexpensive and readily available medication.

Research

In this experiment, the researchers focused on chronic kidney disease and hypertension. The kidneys must balance acids, potassium, and sodium. But with kidney disease, the blood becomes too acidic.

However, in the clinical trials with a daily glass of sodium bicarbonate, not only was acidity reduced, but, most impressively, it slowed the progression of kidney disease!

Daily having a half-to-a-whole teaspoon of baking soda stirred into a glass of warm water reduces the inflammation of autoimmune diseases, according to many scientists researching this subject.

Sodium bicarbonate helps the spleen support an anti-inflammatory environment in preference to the inflammatory disease process that occurs with auto-immune diseases, such as rheumatoid arthritis.

In experiments with both healthy people and rats, it was shown that drinking a solution of sodium bicarbonate triggers the stomach to produce more acid, which helps in digestion. This gets interesting because the mesothelial cells that live on the spleen communicate information in order to mount a protective, anti-inflammatory, immune response.

Mesothelial cells line body cavities, as well as cover the exterior of organs. They have little, one might say finger-like, protrusions, called microvilli. These microvilli read the environment and let the organs that they cover know when there is a need for an immune-inflammatory, theoretically protective, response because of an invader.

However, when one drinks a baking soda mixture, it appears to tell the spleen, which is a blood filter, to temper its immune response. In fact, the spleen, the blood, and the kidneys, with both rat and human participants (medical students recruited for the experiment), shifted M1 macrophages that *promote* inflammation, to M2 macrophages, which *reduce* inflammation, when drinking water with baking soda! In other words, baking soda produced a shift from an inflammatory to an anti-inflammatory response, with not only the kidneys, but also the spleen and the blood, proving to be a safe way to reduce inflammatory disease.

Chapter High Points:

1. Bicarbonate increases the effective impact of several antibiotics against bacteria.

2. Sepsis is a serious problem, with a death rate that exceeds that of breast cancer.

3. Sodium bicarbonate has been shown to support the body when battling against sepsis.

4. When drinking water with baking soda, the spleen, the blood, and the kidneys shift macrophages from M1 to M2 macrophages that reduce inflammation.

5. In ongoing experiments, a daily glass of water with sodium bicarbonate slowed the progression of kidney disease.

6. Baking soda stirred into a glass of warm water has been shown to reduce the inflammation of autoimmune diseases.

7. Reference: https://www.acsh.org/news/2018/01/11/spoonful-baking-soda-helps-antibiotics-go-down-12387

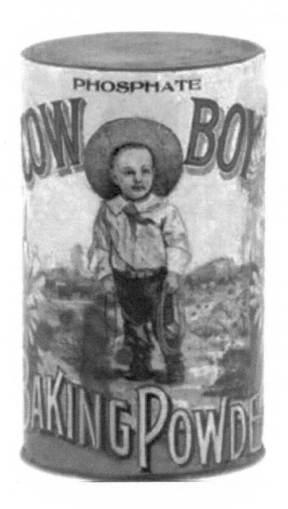

Chapter 8
More Exciting Science About Baking Soda

S odium bicarbonate has many uses due to its ability to react with both acids and bases (alkaline substances).

Sodium bicarbonate is classified as an acid salt, formed by combining an acid (carbonic) and a base (sodium hydroxide), and is a mild alkali in its reaction with other chemicals. Baking soda decomposes into sodium carbonate, which is a more stable substance, water, and carbon dioxide at temperatures above 300 degrees Fahrenheit (149 degrees Celsius).

Baking soda neutralizes odors chemically, rather than masking them.

Carbon dioxide is heavier than air. This action of keeping oxygen can smother flames, which makes sodium bicarbonate useful in fire extinguishers.

Other interesting and scientific applications of sodium bicarbonate include:

Air pollution control – it absorbs sulfur dioxide and other acid gas emissions.

It is used in abrasive blastings for removal of surface coatings.

It precipitates calcium and acts as a lubricant in oil well drilling fluids.

It is used in rubber and plastic manufacturing.

It is used in chemical manufacturing.

It is used in paper manufacturing.

It is used to process textiles.

In the process of water treatment, sodium bicarbonate reduces the level of lead and other heavy metals.

Sodium bicarbonate decomposes into carbon dioxide and water when exposed to a moderately strong acid. This process gives sodium bicarbonate several of its multiple uses.

Sodium Bicarbonate Production

Sodium bicarbonate is produced on a large scale by reacting cold, concentrated brine, sodium chloride, solutions with ammonia and CO_2.

Sodium Bicarbonate Formula

$NaHCO_3$ is the sodium bicarbonate formula. In water this salt, separates into sodium (Na+) cation and carbonate (CO_3-) anions. Typically marketed as a powder, baking soda is an alkaline, white, crystalline substance that tastes a little salty.

Sodium Bicarbonate Properties

The alkaline pH is due to sodium bicarbonate's hydrolysis reaction.

The pH of a sodium bicarbonate solution is between 8-9.5.

It does not entirely dissolve in water.

It has a melting point of 50 degrees Celsius.

The molecular weight is 84.0066 g/mol, which is the molar mass. The molar mass is not a molecular but instead, is a bulk property of a substance.

When it is heated, sodium bicarbonate decomposes and releases carbon dioxide gas, which forms sodium carbonate.

This reaction is what baking soda goes through when heated during cooking.

The Structure of Sodium Bicarbonate, $NaHCO_3$

Baking soda's type of crystal structure is a monoclinic lattice structure. One sodium atom, one carbon atom, one hydrogen atom, and three oxygen atoms make up the structure of baking soda.

Uses of Sodium Bicarbonate

While the science of baking soda has found its way into fireworks, fire extinguishers, fungicides, and pesticides, it may now have new utility for companies looking to improve their environmental footprint as well. *None too soon.*

Future Applications

New research into the science of baking soda is focusing on larger-scale applications of baking soda's cleaning and absorbent properties. In fruit production, it has proved useful removing pesticides from the apples more efficiently than commercial sanitizers. There is chemical degradation of the pesticide when it comes into contact with sodium bicarbonate.

There may also be industrial-scale cleaning potential for coal-fired power plants and other industrial facilities where sodium bicarbonate can be used as a cost-effective solution to neutralize flue gases, in the hopes of both reducing air emissions and generating a marketable product. Sodium bicarbonate can remove up to 99.5 percent of the SO_2 from a smokestack, and is superior to other methods.

National Bicarbonate of Soda Day

Did you know there is a *National Bicarbonate of Soda Day* Which is December 30, for celebrating the science of baking soda? It's appropriately timed when taking into consideration all the baked goods consumed during the holidays and the accompanying indigestion.

This humble salt has a growing list of uses with no sign of diminishing.

Sodium bicarbonate's IUPAC (*International Union of Pure and Applied Chemistry*) name is *Sodium hydrogen carbonate.*

Chapter High Points:

1. Sodium bicarbonate has many uses due to its ability to react with both acids and bases.

2. Sodium bicarbonate is employed in a wide range of manufacturing, including everything from paper and textiles to rubber and chemistry.

3. One sodium atom, one carbon atom, one hydrogen atom, and three oxygen atoms make up sodium bicarbonate.

4. Sodium bicarbonate has significant application in reducing harmful air emissions in industrial facilities.

5. December 30 is the annual *National Bicarbonate of Soda Day!*

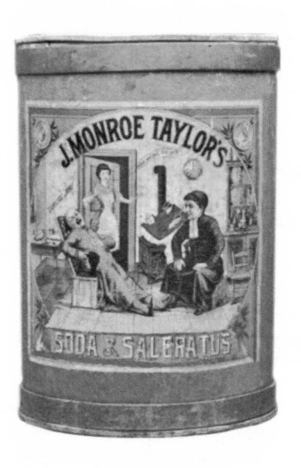

Chapter 9
Cautions and
Possible Side Effects

Internal and external uses of baking soda are generally considered safe and non-toxic. Although oral consumption is safe, don't exceed the recommended dose. The human inclination to think that if a little is good, more is better, needs to be avoided when consuming baking soda.

Bear in mind that this substance has a strong rising action when encountering liquid. A little can be very helpful. A lot can be life-threatening. Think about that beautiful cake in the oven, rising and baking to perfection. If there is too much baking soda in the ingredients, the batter will likely run over the pan and destroy the product. You do not want it taking that sort of action *in you!*

Though seemingly innocent and readily available, too much baking soda can upset the body's pH balance with resulting nausea, vomiting, and/or abdominal pain. Although rare, baking soda overdose can cause seizures, coma, and even death.

Baking soda is quite high in sodium—1,259 milligrams in one teaspoon. Taking high doses is likely to raise blood pressure. It can overload circulation and lead to heart failure. People who consume far too much baking soda have developed blood chemistry imbalances and heart malfunction.

Another reason not to overdo your consumption of baking soda is that it can increase potassium excretion, leading to a potassium deficiency.

If you do take it internally, sip the baking soda and water mixture slowly and remember these points:

Don't drink a baking soda and water mixture in which the baking soda is not fully dissolved.

Don't take more than a tablespoon of baking soda per day.

Don't take the maximum dosage for longer than two weeks.

Don't drink a baking soda solution too quickly.

Don't take it when you're overly full.

Don't take baking soda within two hours of taking other medications.

Don't give baking soda to children under six years of age unless prescribed by the child's pediatrician.

Don't take baking soda internally if you are pregnant or breastfeeding.

Don't take sodium bicarbonate if you have diabetic ketoacidosis, as it raises blood acids known as ketones

Some other products that may interact with baking soda include:
Medications with a coating to protect the stomach
Aspirin and other salicylates
Calcium supplements
Corticosteroids
Barbiturates
Lithium
Quinidine
Diuretics

Also, be aware that it's possible for vitamins, herbal products, prescription drugs, and over-the-counter medicines to interact with baking soda. Put some time between taking supplements and drinking a baking soda beverage.

Please discuss taking baking soda with your trusted healthcare professional if you have edema, liver disease, kidney disease, high blood pressure, if you are on prescription medication, or if you are on a sodium-restricted diet.

Get emergency medical help if a person has the following signs of a serious allergic reaction to the consumption of baking soda:

Hives

Difficulty breathing

Swelling of the face, lips, tongue, or throat

Severe stomach pain

Edema, rapid weight gain

Shortness of breath with mild exertion

Less concerning side effects:

Dry mouth

Increased thirst

Urinating more than usual

Metabolic Alkalosis

Continued excessive use of baking soda may lead to metabolic alkalosis. This is a condition in which the blood becomes overly alkaline, retaining fluids, which does not allow getting rid of the excess bicarbonate ions causing the alkalosis.

Being overly alkaline is as serious as being overly acidic, and can cause heart problems.

Causes of Metabolic Alkalosis

Several conditions can cause metabolic alkalosis, including:

Loss of stomach acids, which is the most common cause of metabolic alkalosis, brought on by vomiting.

Excessive use of antacids. Antacid use won't normally lead to metabolic alkalosis, but in the case of weak or failing kidneys and using a non-absorbable antacid, it can bring on alkalosis.

Diuretics—commonly prescribed for high blood pressure, can cause increased acid in urinary secretion, which can make the blood more alkaline.

Hypokalemia, a potassium deficiency, can cause the hydrogen ions normally present in the fluid around cells to shift to inside the cells. The absence of protective acidic hydrogen ions causes the fluids and blood to become more alkaline.

Effective arterial blood volume (EABV) is reduced due to a weakened heart or cirrhosis of the liver. Reduced blood flow interferes with the body's ability to remove alkaline bicarbonate ions.

And, finally, heart, kidney, or liver failure can lead to potassium depletion.

Symptoms of Metabolic Alkalosis

Slow breathing

Fast or irregular heartbeats, dizziness, or lightheadedness

Blue skin or nails

Confusion or feeling irritable

Muscle cramps or spasms

Trouble breathing

Sodium bicarbonate includes salt and can raise the risk of edema

High blood calcium levels may cause difficulty excreting bicarbonate

Baking soda can reduce blood potassium levels. Avoid it if you already have low levels of potassium

Sodium bicarbonate reduces the amount of iron absorbed by the body. Take sodium bicarbonate and iron supplements separately if you are iron deficient.

Chapter High Points:

1. It is possible to upset the body's pH and become too alkaline. Do not exceed the recommended dosage of baking soda.

2. Keep in mind that baking soda is quite high in sodium.

3. Become familiar with the products and medications that may interact with baking soda.

4. The most significant high point of this chapter: *All Things in Moderation!*

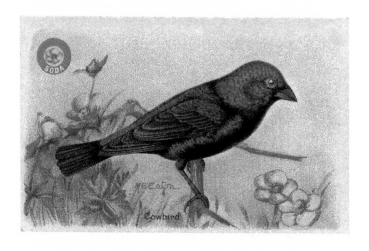

Cowbird

Medical Disclaimer

Although this book is based on recent scientific research, the content should not be considered as medical advice or a recommendation for medical treatment. This content is strictly educational and informational. Readers are strongly recommended to consult with their healthcare professional regarding health issues and treatments.

My Gift for You ....

Thank you for reading **Save Your Life with Basic Baking Soda.** I have a gift for you:

Save Your Life with Stupendous Spices.

To receive your ebook, type in the following link:

https://BookHip.com/DKHVDA

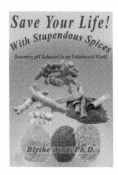

About the Author ....

I live in the midst (and often the mist) of ten acres of forest, with domestic and wild creatures, where I create an ever-growing inventory of self-help, health, and meditation nonfiction books, novels, short stories, and illustrated kid's books, along with quite a bit of poetry. I've also begun audio recording my books.

I do a bit of wood carving when I need a change of pace, and I'm frequently on a ladder, cleaning my gutters. It's spectacular being on a ladder ... the vista opens up all around, and I feel rather like a bird or a squirrel, perched on a metal branch.

After I received my Doctorate from the University of California at Irvine in the School of Social Sciences, (majoring in psychology and ethnography), I moved to the Pacific Northwest to write and to have a modest private psychotherapy practice in a small town not much bigger than a village.

Finally, I decided it was time to put my full focus on my writing, where, through the world-shrinking internet, I could "meet" greater numbers of people. *Where I could meet you!*

All the creatures in my forest and I are glad you "stopped by." If you enjoyed **Save Your Life with Basic Baking Soda**, I hope you'll share the book with others. If you want to write to me, I'd love to hear from you.

Here's my email:

Blythe@BlytheAyne.com

And here's my website:

www.BlytheAyne.com

And my *Boutique of Books*:

https://shop.BlytheAyne.com

I hope to "see" you again!

Blythe

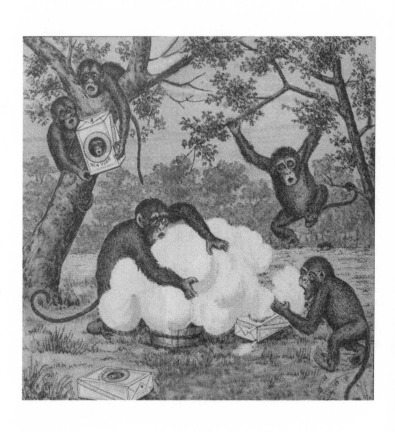

GLOSSARY:

Acidic - pH below 7.

Alkaline - pH greater than 7.

Allergens - Substances causing allergic reactions.

Antibiotic - A substance that inhibits the growth of or destroys microorganisms.

Antibodies - Blood proteins that combine with substances the body recognizes as alien such as bacteria, viruses, and foreign substances in the blood to destroy them.

Antibacterial - A substance or process that is active against bacteria.

Anti-fungal - A substance or process that is active against fungus.

Antihistamine - A compound for treating allergies that inhibits the effects of histamine.

Anti-inflammatory - Used to reduce inflammation.

Antioxidants - A substance such as vitamin C or E that removes potentially damaging oxidizing agents in a living organism.

Antiseptic - Substances that prevent the growth of disease-causing microorganisms.

Antiviral - A substance or process that is effective against viruses

Apo B - The structural protein of the LDL cholesterol molecule.

Cholesterol - A sterol compound found in most body tissues including blood and nerves. Cholesterol and its derivatives are important components of cell membranes.

    HDL - good - high-density lipoprotein that removes cholesterol from the blood. It is associated with a reduced risk of atherosclerosis and heart disease.

    LDL - bad - the form of lipoprotein in which cholesterol is transported in the blood.

Enzymes - Catalysts to specific biochemical reactions. Most enzymes are proteins of large, complex molecule

Hypertension - High blood pressure.

Lactic acid - A colorless organic acid formed in sour milk and produced in muscle tissues during strenuous exercise.

Nutrients - Any substance, such as protein, vitamins, or minerals that provides nourishment for the growth and maintenance of life.

pH Scale - A scale measuring from one, extremely acidic, to fourteen, extremely alkaline.

pH Balance - A balanced pH is near 7.365 on the pH scale.

Toxins - Harmful chemicals.

Uric Acid - Derived from purines. When uric acid crystallizes it becomes gout.

Uricase - A digestive enzyme that breaks down purines.

Proteins - Nitrogenous organic compounds consisting of large molecules, composed of one or more long chains of amino acids.

URLs and References:

https://www.acsh.org/news/2018/01/11/spoonful-baking-soda-helps-antibiotics-go-down-12387

https://naturalremedyideas.com/12-amazing-health-benefits-of-baking-soda/

https://draxe.com/nutrition/baking-soda-uses/

https://www.epicnaturalhealth.com/29-benefits-of-drinking-baking-soda-water/

https://www.healthline.com/nutrition/baking-soda-benefits-uses#household-uses

https://www.crystalhills.com/history-and-use-of-sodium-bicarbona

https://www.linkedin.com/pulse/sodium-bicarbonate-discovery-production-uses-rita-martin/

benjaminbarber.org. 08 2019. 01 2023. https://benjaminbarber.org/history-of-baking-soda/

https://sodiumbicarbonate.net/uses-of-sodium-bicarbonate/

https://www.atlasobscura.com/articles/baking-soda-history

https://www.primidi.com/sodium_bicarbonate/history

https://www.primidi.com/slc4a5

https://www.wellandgood.com/why-to-drink-baking-soda/

https://www.healthykidneyclub.com › is-baking-soda-safe-for-kidney-disease

https://worldhistory.us/ancient-history/ancient-egypt/ancient-egypt-beauty-makeup-and-hygiene.php

https://www.madsci.org/posts/archives/2000-11/975608559.Sh.r.html

https://circle.adventistlearningcommunity.com/download/LittleHouseSSUnit.pdf\

https://axial.acs.org/2018/08/03/the-science-of-baking-soda/

https://benjaminbarber.org/

https://www.turito.com/blog/chemistry/sodium-bicarbonate

https://fdc.nal.usda.gov/fdc-app.html#/food-details/175040/nutrients

https://pubmed.ncbi.nlm.nih.gov/32651702/

https://www.ncbi.nlm.nih.gov/books/NBK559139/

https://pubmed.ncbi.nlm.nih.gov/24313600/

https://www.ncbi.nlm.nih.gov/books/NBK279254/

https://www.tandfonline.com/doi/abs/10.3810/psm.1998.07.1617?journalCode=ipsm20

https://www.ncbi.nlm.nih.gov/pmc/articles/PMC100914/

https://pubmed.ncbi.nlm.nih.gov/6990140/

Industrial:

https://cen.acs.org/articles/88/i24/Familiar-Product-Different-Use.html?utm_source=pcm&utm_medium=axial&utm_campaign=PUBS_0322_FJG_baking_soda&src=PUBSaxial_baking_soda

Exercise:

https://www.ncbi.nlm.nih.gov/pmc/articles/PMC4475610/

https://pubmed.ncbi.nlm.nih.gov/27399820/

Sodium bicarb as Ergogenic Aid

https://www.ncbi.nlm.nih.gov/pmc/articles/PMC5059234/

https://pubmed.ncbi.nlm.nih.gov/25494054/

https://pubmed.ncbi.nlm.nih.gov/34503527/

Renal:

https://www.ncbi.nlm.nih.gov/books/NBK538339/

https://pubmed.ncbi.nlm.nih.gov/30220653/

https://pubmed.ncbi.nlm.nih.gov/24107852/

https://pubmed.ncbi.nlm.nih.gov/25606047/

https://circle.adventistlearningcommunity.com/download/LittleHouseSSUnit.pdf

https://www.eatingwell.com/article/7825078/baking-soda-uses-cleaning-cooking/

https://www.eatingwell.com/article/14576/the-weird-reason-you-should-be-adding-baking-soda-to-your-beans/

https://www.ncbi.nlm.nih.gov/pmc/articles/PMC4475610/

Baking Soda and UTIs:

https://pubmed.ncbi.nlm.nih.gov/28975365/

Baking Soda and Kids Creativity:

https://homegrownfriends.com/home/multi-sensory-baking-soda-vinegar-experiment/

Kiefer, David M. Soda ash, Solvay style writer

OECD SIDS. Sodium Bicarbonate (accessed 05 February 2018).

Development of Baking Powder: National Historic Chemical Landmark.

Science Service. J Chem Ed 1927;4 (12):1492.

Farha et al. ACS Infect Dis 2017; DOI: 10.1021/acsinfecdis.7b00194.

Yang et al. J Agric Food Chem 2017;65:9744–9752

Pittman. Chem Eng News 2010;88(24):34.

Chem Eng News, Pittman 2010;88(24):34

Chem Eng News, Johnson 2014;92(46):26–27

https://images.acspubs.org/EloquaImages/clients/AmericanChemicalSociety/{2c75a536-fbdd-4c64-a2ee-f7ed-b435d953}_ACS-Publications-Periodic-Table-2020.png

https://www.drugs.com/mtm/sodium-bicarbonate.html

Baking Soda – How Products Are Made, Sideman, Eva 1994 Encyclopedia. com.

http://www. encyclopedia. com/doc/1G2-2896500017

html BookRags Staff. "Baking Soda" 2005 (September 20, 2010)

http://www. bookrags. com/research/baking-soda-woi

How was sodium bicarbonate discovered, Fellows, Chris 2000

http://www. madsci. org/posts/archives/2000-11/975608559

Made in the USA
Coppell, TX
31 January 2024

28456506R00069